WHAT'S FOR DINNER

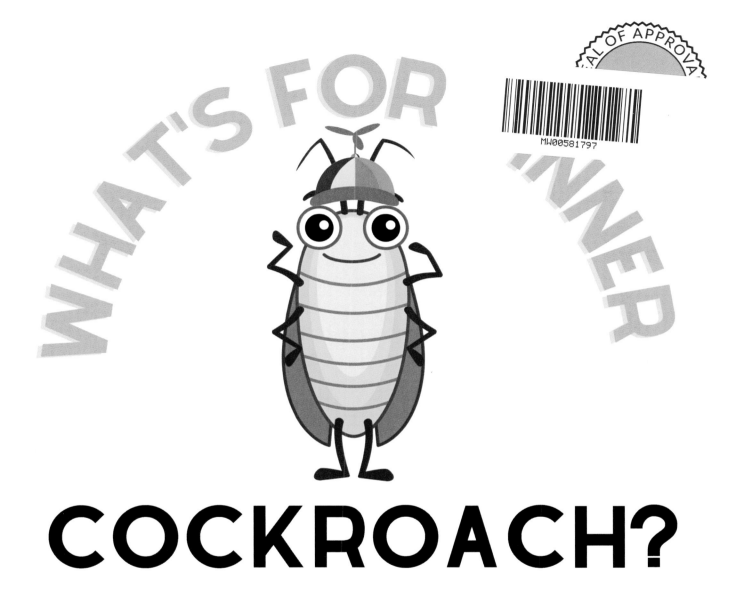

COCKROACH?

A children's book about supportive meal environments

By Kelly Picard PhD RD

Illustrations created using Canva

Author's note

I wrote this book to demonstrate what supportive meal time environments look like.

As the week goes by, note that Cockroach is offered a variety of foods, some that he normally enjoys and some that he isn't sure about. Also note that the adults trust him and his body to know what the right amount of food is for him at each meal. They do this without offering praise or reprimand, regardless of his choices at meal time.

- His caregivers are in charge of what is offered and when.
- Cockroach is in charge of whether or not to eat and how much.

For Chris, Walter and Oscar

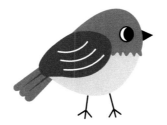

On Monday, Cockroach's Dea served worms, dung and flies for dinner.

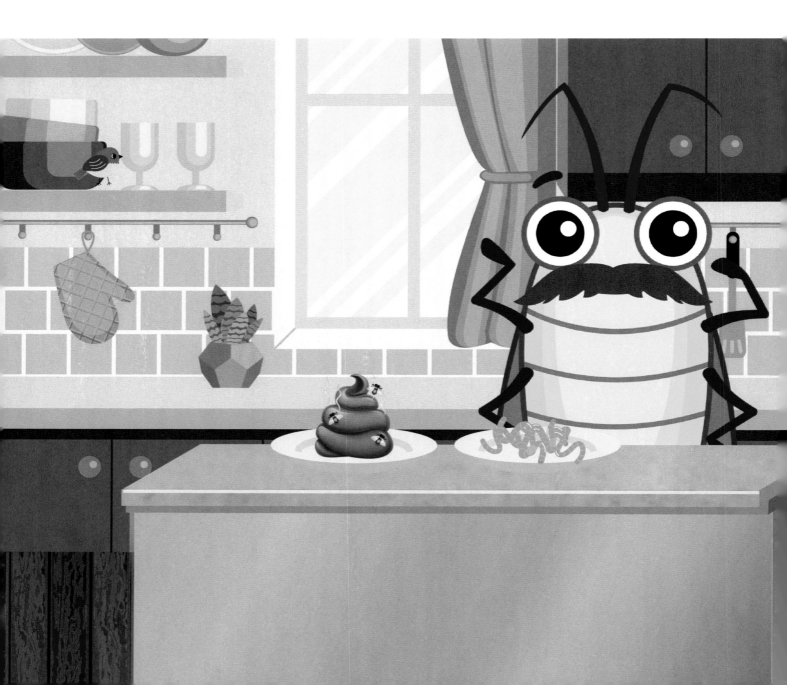

Normally, Cockroach ate worms, dung and flies for dinner. BUT...

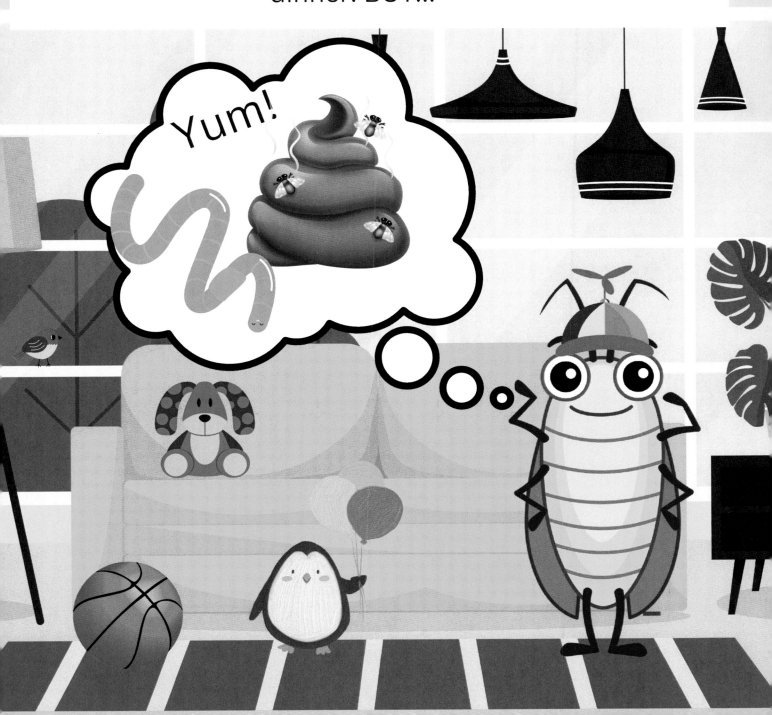

Today Cockroach wasn't feeling very hungry. After eating 2 flies and 1 worm, Cockroach said "I'm full."

Dea didn't say anything about how much or how little Cockroach ate.

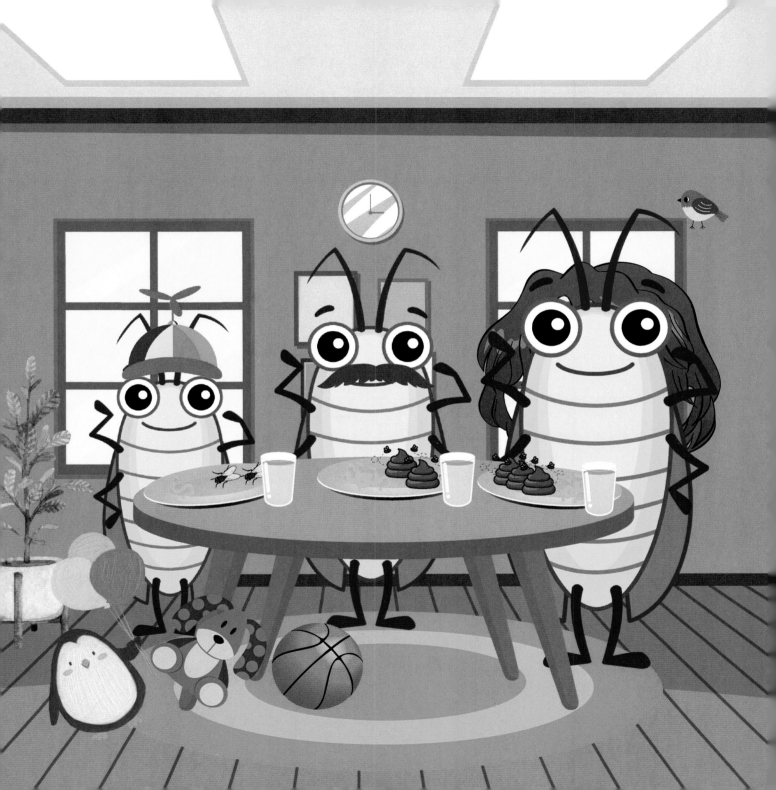

The next day was Tuesday. Cockroach's Blatto served grass clippings, soggy leaves and rotten meat for dinner.

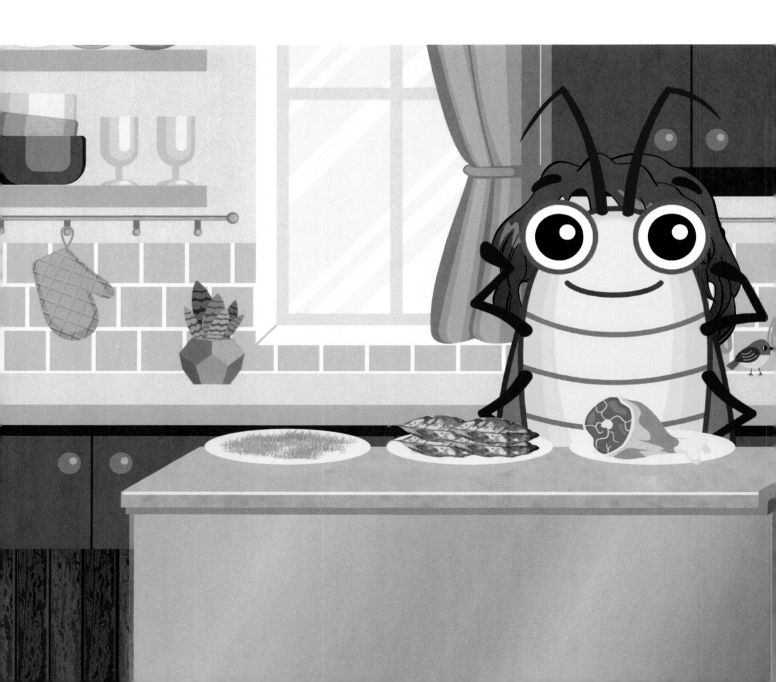

Normally, Cockroach ate grass clippings, soggy leaves and rotten meat for dinner, BUT...

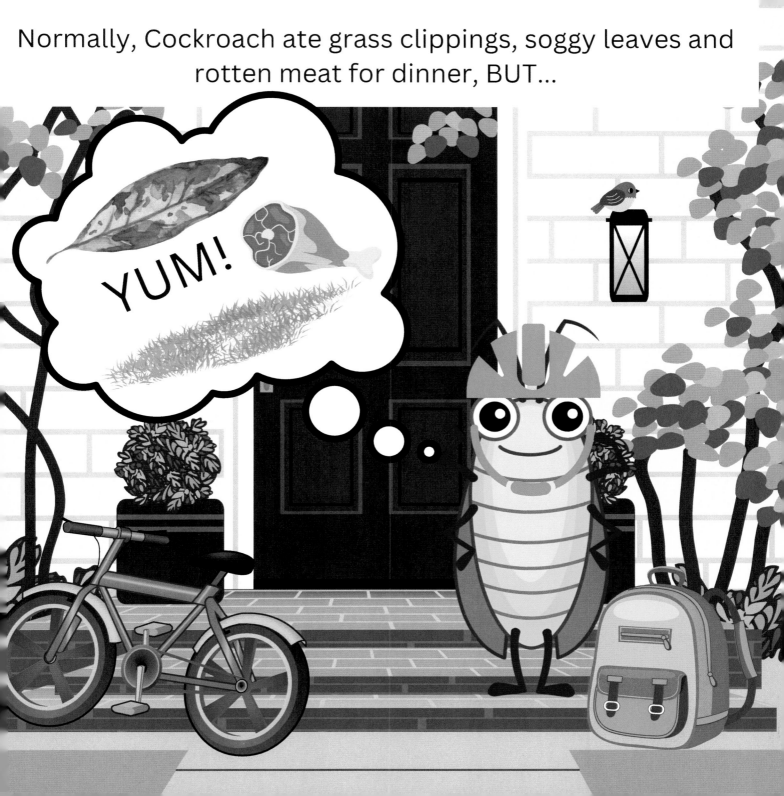

Today Cockroach felt more like talking about his bike ride than eating dinner. After eating 2 blades of grass, half a soggy leaf and 1 bite of rotten meat, Cockroach said "I'm full."

Blatto didn't say anything about how much or how little Cockroach ate.

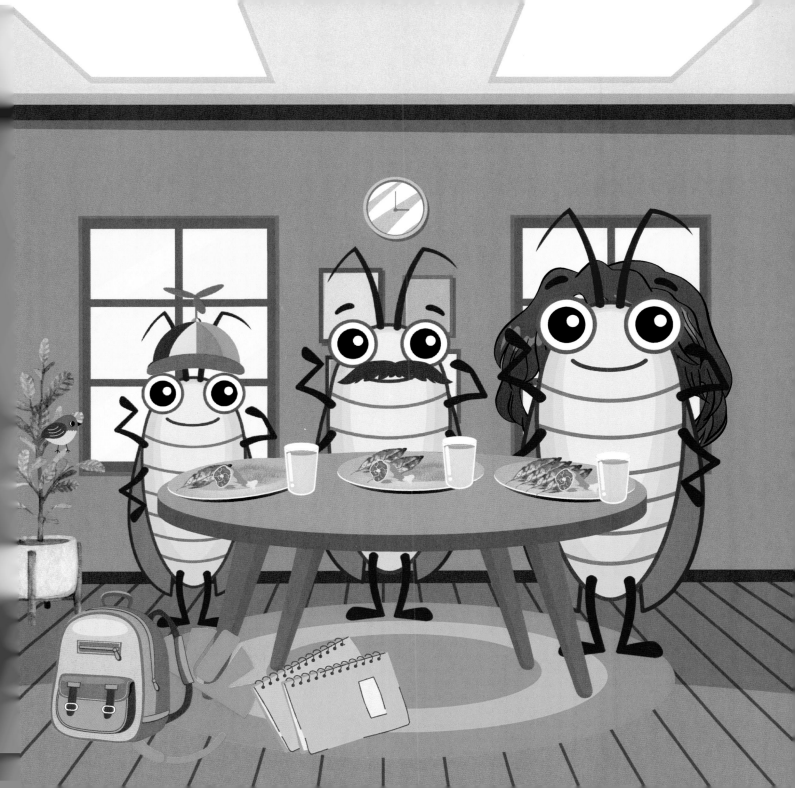

The next day was Wednesday. Cockroach's Dea served moldy bread, slimy watermelon rinds and stinky steaks for dinner.

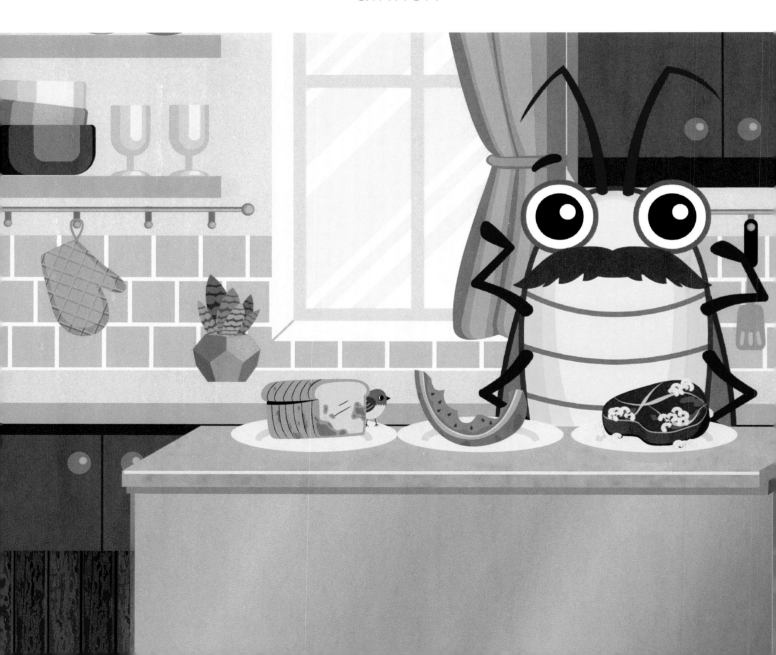

Normally, Cockroach ate moldy bread, slimy watermelon rinds and stinky steaks for dinner. BUT...

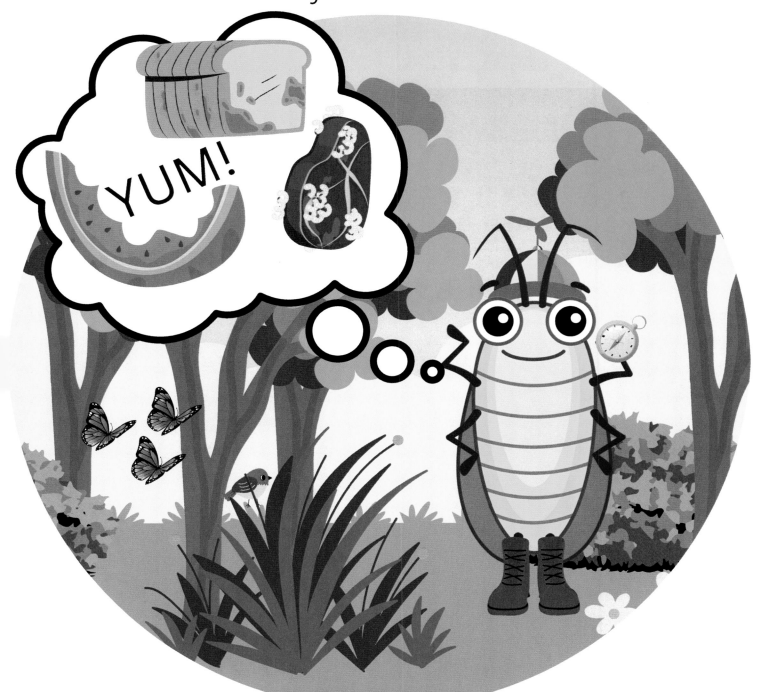

Today Cockroach was feeling tired from walking in the woods. After eating 3 bites of moldy bread, 4 bites of slimy watermelon and no stinky steak, Cockroach said "I'm full."

Dea didn't say anything about how much or how little Cockroach ate.

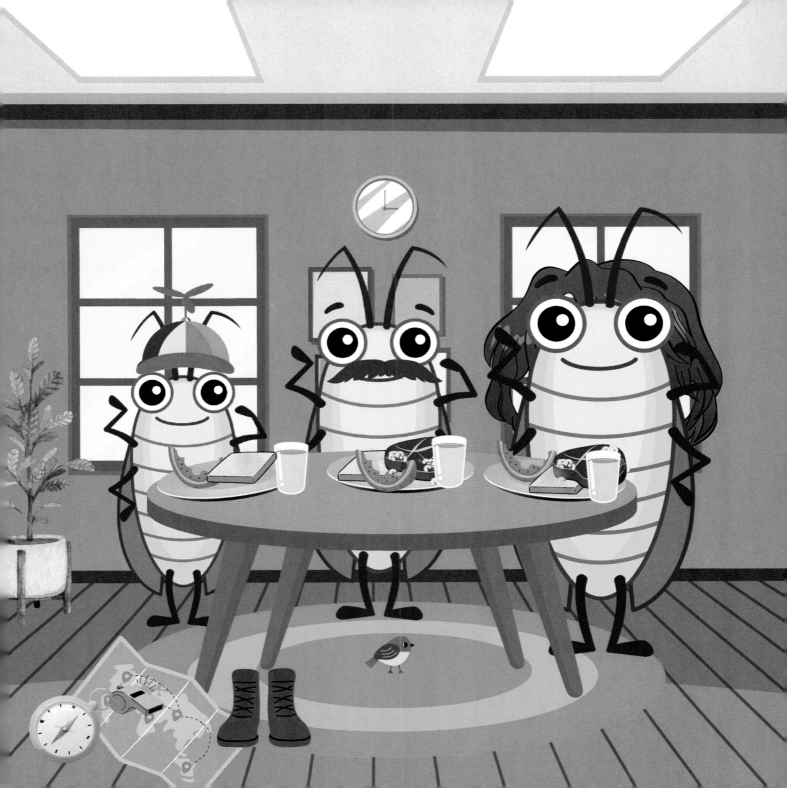

The next day was Thursday. Cockroach's Blatto served wormy apples, fuzzy mold wedges and ear wax curls for dinner.

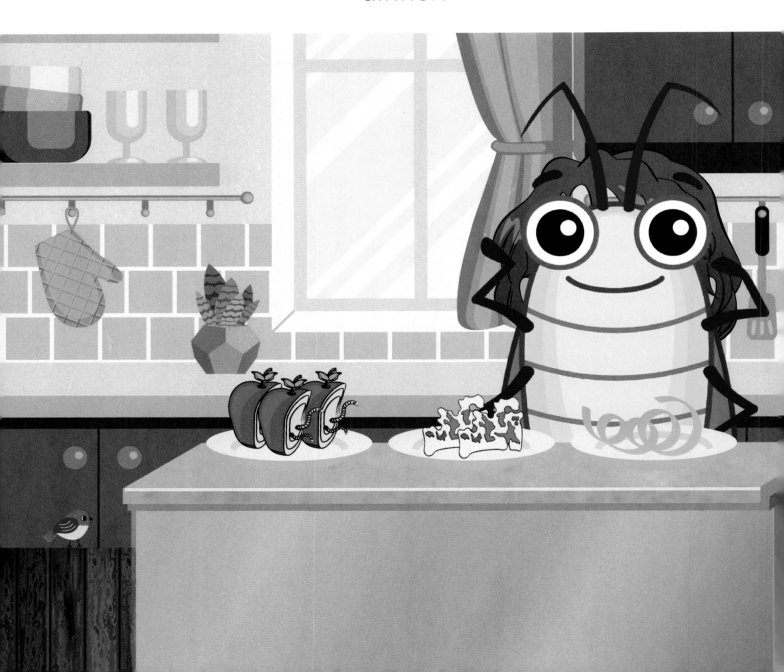

Normally, Cockroach ate wormy apples, fuzzy mold wedges and ear wax curls for dinner. BUT...

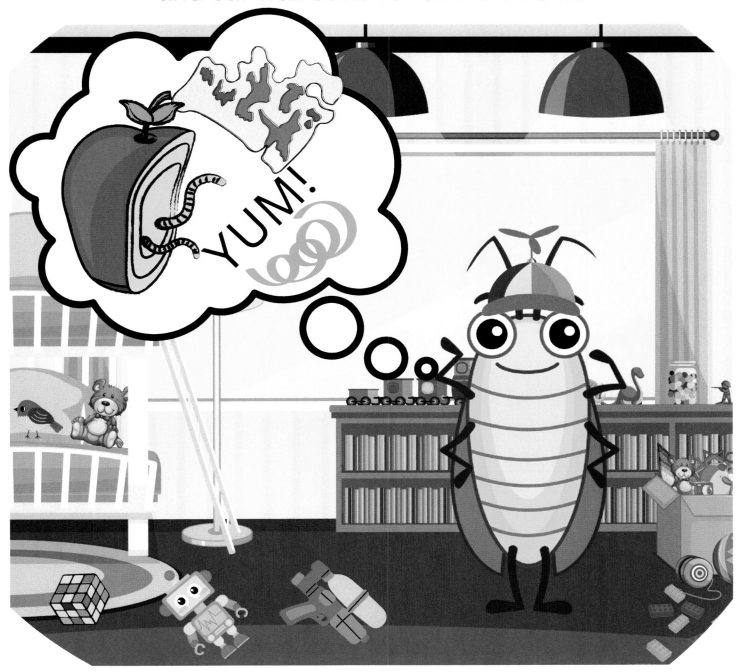

Today Cockroach had a sore tummy. After eating 1 wormy apple but no fuzzy mold wedges or ear wax curls, Cockroach said "I'm full."

Blatto didn't say anything about how much or how little Cockroach ate.

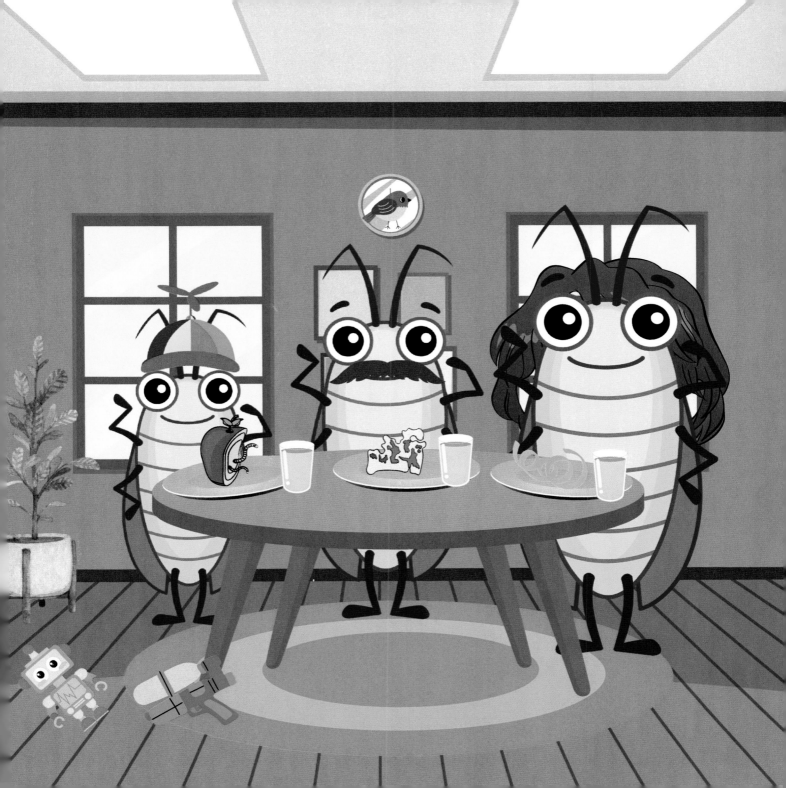

The next day was Friday. Cockroach's Dea served cow patties, bruised bananas and rotten eggs WITH shells!

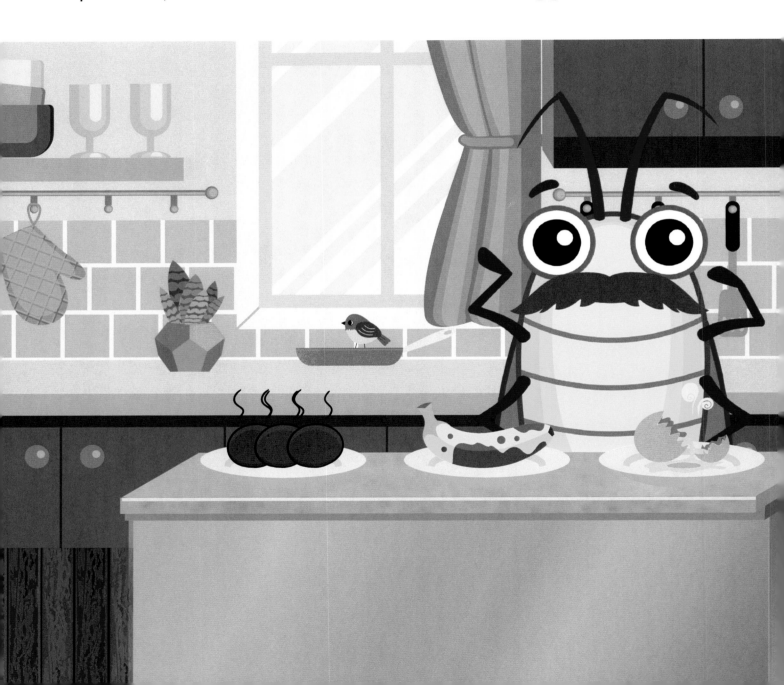

Cockroach knew he enjoyed cow patties. He wasn't sure about bruised bananas and rotten eggs with shells. BUT...

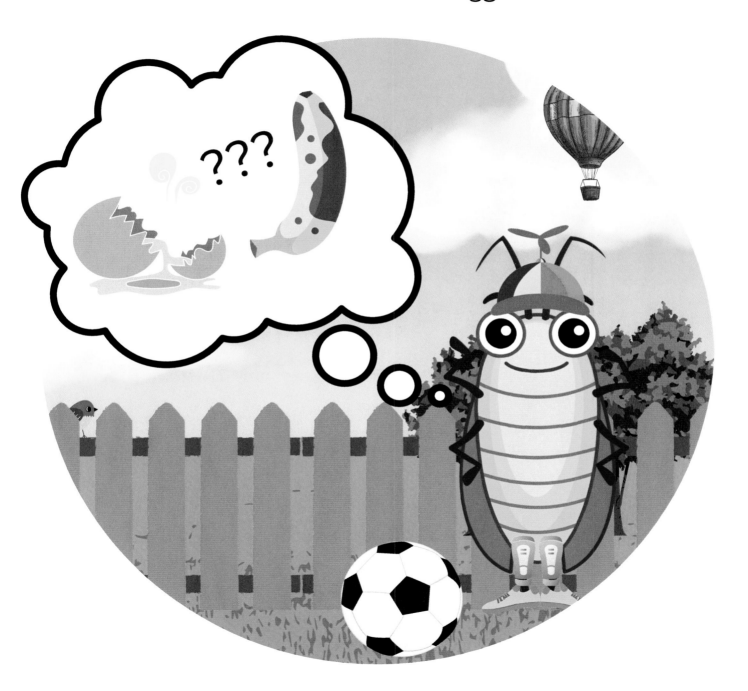

Today Cockroach was feeling adventurous. After eating 2 cow patties, Cockroach decided to try the eggs and bananas. Cockroach ate 3 eggs and 4 bruised bananas, then said "I'm full."

Dea didn't say anything about how much or how little Cockroach ate.

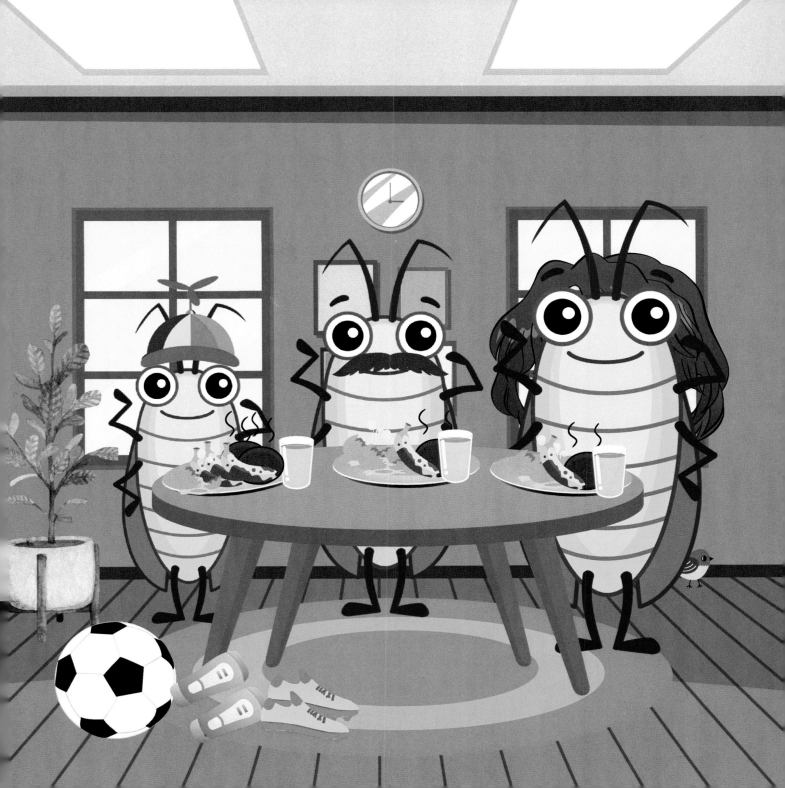

The next day was Saturday. Cockroach's Blatto served giant octopus toes, swamp sludge and Dea's mustache clippings for dinner.

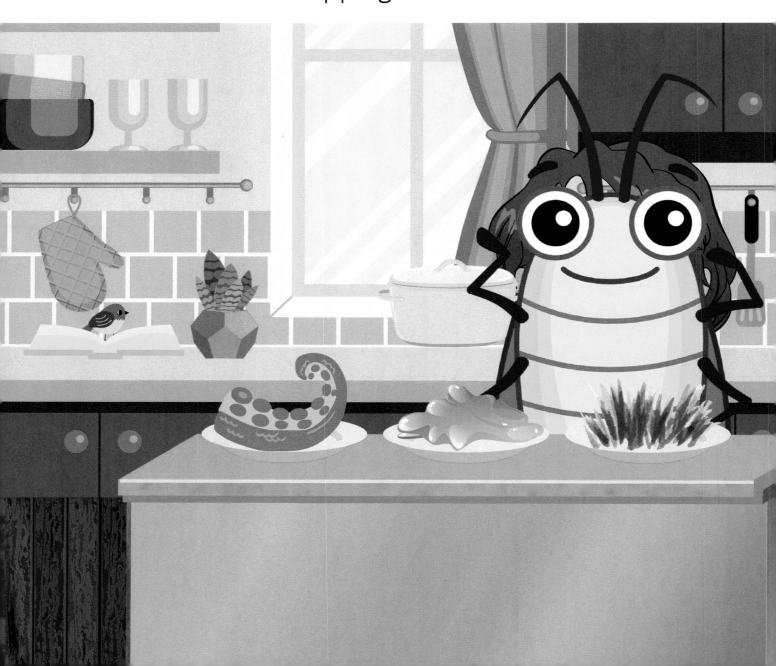

Cockroach was hoping for melted ice cream that had fallen in the sand for dinner. BUT...

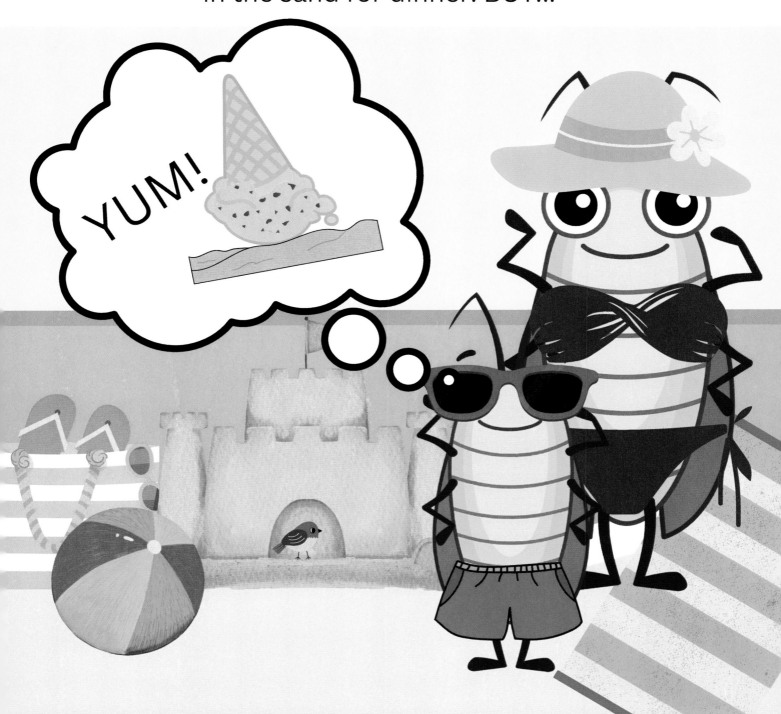

Cockroach ate 1 bite of Octopus toes and said "That tastes SO good!"

Cockroach ate 4 more octopus toes, 5 scoops of swamp sludge but no mustache clippings.
Then Cockroach said "I'm full."

Blatto didn't say anything about how much or how little Cockroach ate.

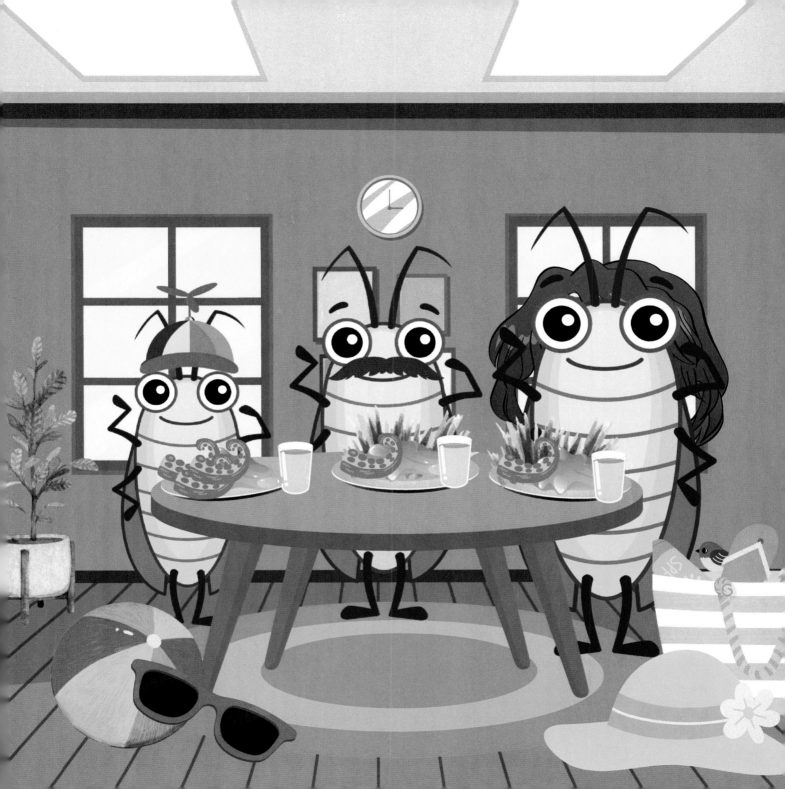

The next day was Sunday. Cockroach's Dea and Blatto served their family's super, special, stinky dinner of garbage salad, sludgy worm pudding and rotten cheese for dinner.

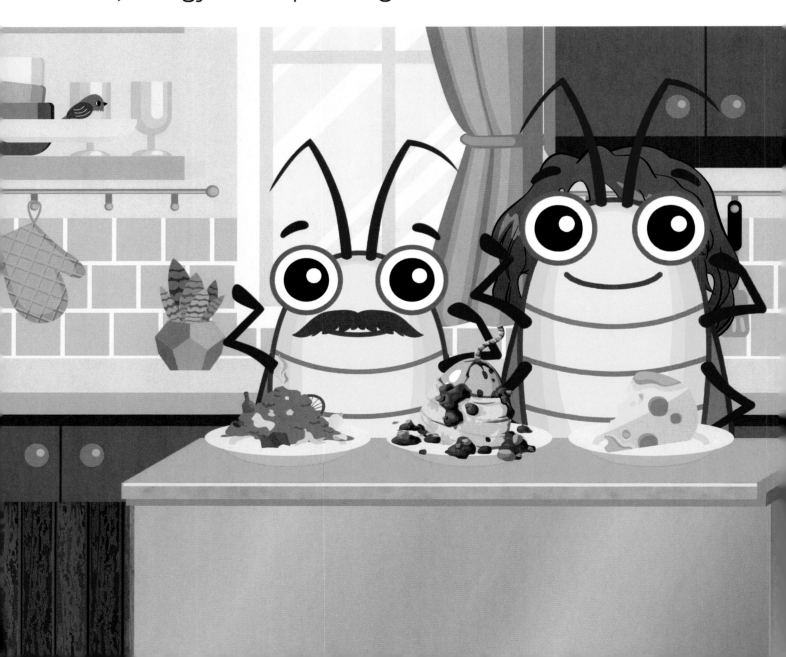

Cockroach had been hoping for pizza that had been sitting in the garbage bin for a few days. BUT...

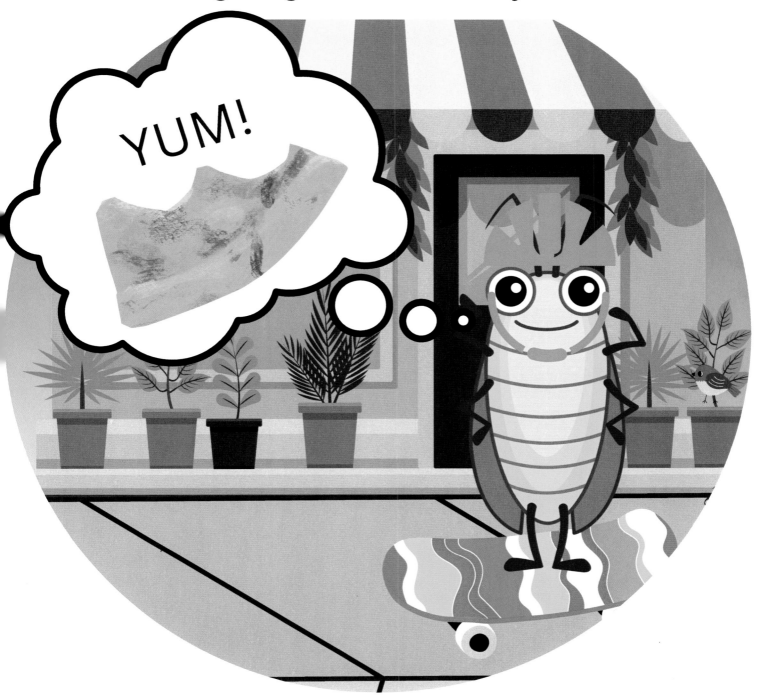

Today Cockroach was hungry. After eating 4 scoops of garbage salad, 5 scoops of sludgy worm pudding and 6 pieces of rotten cheese, Cockroach said "I'm full."

Neither Dea or Blatto said anything about how much or how little Cockroach ate.

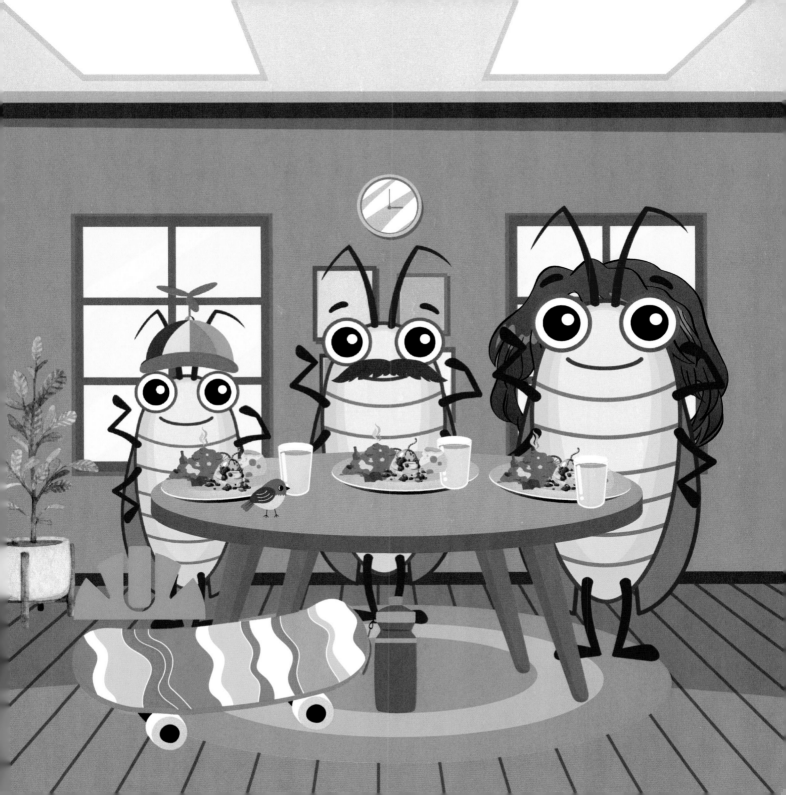

The next day was Monday...

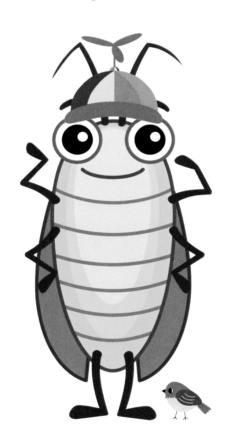

Fun Facts About Cockroaches

The scientific name for cockroaches is Blattodea

Cockroaches are omnivores

Cockroaches are social

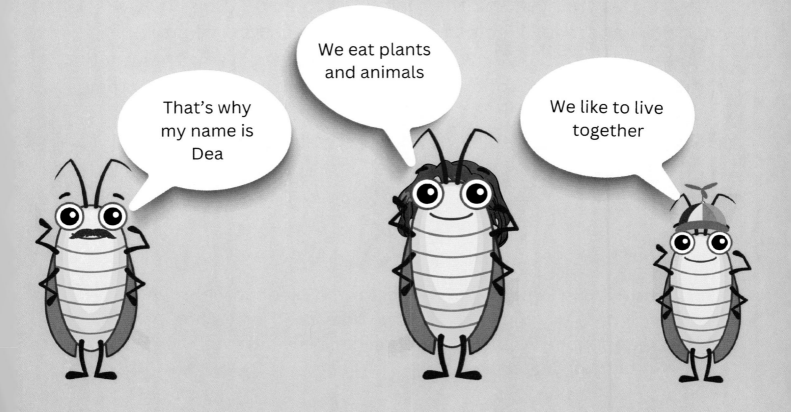

A note for parents: At times, it's normal to worry about how much children eat at meal times. However it is normal for children to eat more on some days and less on other days.

As adults, our job is to choose when foods are offered, choose which foods to offer and trust our children to do their jobs. Our children's job is to decide whether or not to eat from what is offered and how much.

Trusting our children and their instincts to guide them in how much to eat at meals helps them develop positive relationships with food, learn to try new foods in a safe space, grow the way that nature has intended for them and learn how to enjoy family meals.

Find more resources at: https://www.ellynsatterinstitute.org/

About the Author: Kelly Picard is a Registered Dietitian with a PhD in nutrition. She is also the mother of two boys - and knows how hard it can be to create supportive meal environments. Kelly lives with her family in British Columbia, Canada.

Manufactured by Amazon.ca
Bolton, ON

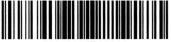

37658156R00021